TABLE OF CONTENTS

CHAIR YOGA FOR SENIORS OVER 60

10 Minutes a Day to Enhance Flexibility, Balance, and Mobility - A Quick and Simple Step-by-Step Guide for Weight Loss and Improved Independence

ARNOLD BARBER

INTRODUCTION:

The benefits of practicing yoga are truly endless, and they become even more pronounced as we age. If you are an aging adult, incorporating yoga into your daily routine can bring about a multitude of advantages that enhance your overall well-being. From increased flexibility and mobility to improved balance and memory, yoga offers a holistic approach to maintaining and improving physical and mental health. As we get older, our bodies undergo various changes that can affect our physical abilities and overall health. Decreased flexibility, weakened muscles, and increased susceptibility to chronic health issues can make it challenging to engage in regular yoga practice. Traditional yoga poses on a mat may seem intimidating or even unattainable for individuals with physical limitations or pre-existing conditions like osteoarthritis, chronic pain, or cardiovascular problems. Fortunately, there is an accessible and gentle alternative that enables individuals to experience the advantages of yoga without the physical demands of traditional poses.

Chair yoga provides a safe and effective means of practicing yoga while being seated or temporarily standing with support. It is a modified form of yoga that adapts traditional poses to accommodate individuals with limited mobility, balance issues, or other physical challenges. You can embark on a transformative journey of chair yoga by utilizing a stable chair, a flat surface, and a basic understanding of the practice. Chair yoga is a versatile practice that can be modified in order to meet your personal needs and abilities. It incorporates a combination of gentle stretches, modified yoga poses, breathing exercises, and relaxation techniques. The practice can be tailored to address specific areas of concern, such as joint mobility, core strength, or stress reduction.

Whether you are new to yoga or an experienced practitioner, chair yoga offers a welcoming and inclusive environment for all. By dedicating just ten short minutes of your day to chair yoga exercises, you can experience a significant improvement in your quality of life. The chair yoga practice offers a wide range of physical and mental benefits. It can help increase your range of motion and flexibility, improve muscle strength and tone, enhance balance and stability, and promote better posture. Chair yoga also stimulates circulation, aids digestion, and supports overall cardiovascular health.

Additionally, the practice can reduce stress, anxiety, and depression, leading to improved mental well-being and a greater sense of calm and inner peace. Chair yoga is especially beneficial for aging adults, creating a safe and comfortable environment to nurture physical and emotional well-being. As we age, it becomes increasingly important to maintain flexibility, mobility, and strength to support independence and overall health. Chair yoga offers a low-impact form of exercise that minimizes the risk of injury while providing numerous benefits. The practice can help combat the effects of sedentary lifestyles and promote an active and vibrant approach to aging.

In this comprehensive and user-friendly guide, created by me, Arnold Barber, a long-time yoga practitioner, you will gain a wealth of knowledge about chair yoga. Having devoted years to the practice of yoga, I am deeply passionate about sharing the wonders of this ancient healing art. Through my experiences, I have witnessed firsthand the remarkable benefits of yoga to my students and myself.

While I have enjoyed numerous physical benefits, such as improved flexibility and balance, it is the profound sense of peace and tranquility that I have achieved through yoga that truly enriches my life. Without this practice, my life would not be as fulfilling as it is today. Throughout my yoga journey, I have explored both traditional mat yoga and chair yoga, and I have discovered that chair yoga is exceptionally accessible to a wide range of people. I firmly believe that everyone should have the opportunity to experience the transformative benefits of yoga, regardless of age or physical condition. This belief has fueled my desire to write this book and share my chair yoga knowledge.

Within the pages of this book, you will find detailed instructions, accompanied by illustrations, on how to enhance your flexibility, balance, and mobility through the practice of chair yoga. From gentle stretches and seated poses to breathing exercises and relaxation techniques, you will be guided through a variety of practices that can be easily incorporated into your daily routine. The step-by-step instructions, combined with insights into the philosophy and principles of yoga, will empower you to embark on a fulfilling and beneficial chair yoga practice. In addition to the physical benefits, chair yoga also nurtures mental well-being. Chair yoga allows for a profound connection between the mind and body by focusing on the breath and engaging in mindful movement. The practice promotes relaxation, stress reduction, and increased mindfulness, which can have a transformative effect on your overall outlook and emotional state. With chair yoga, you will discover a sanctuary of peace and self-care that is always accessible to you, no matter your circumstances. The practice of chair yoga can provide a sense of grounding and stability, allowing you to cultivate resilience and inner strength as you navigate the challenges that come with aging. As you remain consistent with this practice and advance, you will gain a deep sense of confidence and trust in yourself. I do want to remind you to take this one step at a time and be gentle with yourself as you learn about this practice and integrate it into your life.

It is my sincerest hope that this book will serve as a valuable resource on your journey toward improved health and well-being. Whether you are a senior over 60 seeking to maintain your vitality or an individual facing physical limitations due to injury or disability, chair yoga offers a path for you to experience the incredible benefits of this ancient practice. Together, let us embrace the power of chair yoga and unlock the potential for a more vibrant, balanced, and fulfilling life. By integrating chair yoga into your daily routine, you can amplify your mental and physical well-being, cultivate a greater sense of self-awareness, and experience the transformative effects of this ancient practice. I invite you to embark on this journey with me, and I am confident that chair yoga will bring about positive changes in your life that will ripple through all aspects of your being. So, take a seat, find comfort in your chair, and let the transformative practice of chair yoga unfold before you. Your body, mind, and spirit will thank you.

CHAPTER 1:

UNDERSTANDING CHAIR YOGA.

Traditional yoga is an ancient healing practice that originated in India and has been around for over 5,000 years. It promotes holistic well-being through spiritual, mental, and physical practices. This practice involves physical postures known as asanas, breathing techniques known as pranayama, and meditations known as dhyana. Being derived from traditional yoga, chair yoga was founded by yoga therapist Lakshmi Voelker during the early 1980s. One of Voelker's yoga students was diagnosed with arthritis and was no longer able to practice yoga on the floor due to physical limitations. Determined to help her student out and create an alternative, she developed a yoga sequence for her student to practice on a chair. Ever since then, she has trained and certified thousands of teachers. Students in their late 70s with many neck and back surgeries told they could never practice yoga again were able to reconnect to this practice through chair yoga. Voelker herself was diagnosed with osteopenia, a condition that weakens bones, a few years after inventing chair yoga. She rejected medications for this condition and instead built a chair yoga practice that would build her muscle mass and combat this condition. After months of consistent practice, she had a bone mass test completed and discovered that she did not have osteopenia anymore. She was healed through her chair yoga practice.

If you struggle with low flexibility, balance issues, limitations with mobility, poor weight management, chronic pain, or poor mental health, chair yoga could be just the intervention you need to improve your life. With aging, it can be frustrating to feel like you have to depend on others. Whether it's your inability to take a walk around the block or struggles with independently handling personal hygiene, physical limitations of any degree can make your daily life challenging. While it may seem like things will only go downhill as we age, this does not have to be true for you. There are various ways to reduce the adverse effects that aging can have on our mental and physical health. Chair yoga is one of the best interventions to improve the issues mentioned above, and it is a feasible and accessible practice for anyone. No matter how old you are or how many ailments you are struggling with, you can get started on this practice with ease and experience an abundance of benefits from doing so. Chair yoga was specifically created so that this beautiful healing practice could be accessible to anyone. This practice is ideal for anyone but is especially beneficial for seniors over 60, individuals with physical limitations, or those recovering from injuries. With that being said, let's dive deeper into what chair yoga actually is.

When you think of yoga, what do you imagine? Headstands, backbends, or other crazy balancing acts? While this may reflect super-advanced floor yoga, it is important to realize that yoga comes in various forms and levels of difficulty. There's no need to worry because we will not get into these intense and daunting practices. Chair yoga is significantly simpler and safer, making it an amazing option for older adults, seniors, or individuals who require more stability during their practice. Chair yoga is a safe and gentle practice that involves doing yoga poses while seated or temporarily standing with support. The traditional yoga poses are modified in a way that allows them to be performed while sitting or temporarily standing, depending on your needs. I want to reassure you that there is no need to do intense and challenging poses in a scorching hot studio to experience the perks of yoga! All that you need to begin this practice is a stable chair, a flat surface, and a basic understanding of the practice (which you will gain through reading this book).

A yoga chair is the main tool that will be used during this practice. A yoga chair typically looks like a foldable metal chair that is quite sturdy. It may have an empty space in the back which allows you to practice more advanced poses. You may be thinking, do I have to order a special chair? The short answer is no. While there are multiple different options to choose from online, a chair that you have at home is adequate. As long as it is sturdy and has all of the features that promote safety, then you can use any chair. Some of the most important features to look for in a yoga chair are that it has a sturdy frame, a wide seat, and a backrest. The only downside to not using an actual yoga chair is that it can limit the number of poses you can do. However, as a beginner, you can absolutely start with any sturdy chair you have at home.

One of the best parts of chair yoga is that regardless of your age or any physical limitations, it is fully possible to practice it on a daily basis. As we discussed earlier, students with multiple surgeries and difficult conditions have been able to practice chair yoga. This practice shows us that maintaining a healthy lifestyle does not have to end once we hit age 60 or when we begin to experience physical limitations. The beauty of this practice is that it can be modified so that it can meet your specific needs and abilities. For instance, if you prefer performing solely seated poses, you can choose to only incorporate these ones into your daily practice. If you feel like you are ready for more of a challenge and feel stable, you can incorporate supported standing poses into your practice. The aspects of mindfulness and meditation can also be curated to your liking. You can choose where your attention goes and whether or not you'd like to close your eyes. There are also various breathing techniques that we will later discuss that you can choose from. And, of course, you have the freedom to do it for as long as you'd like to, but just 10 minutes a day is enough to experience the benefits of this practice. There is no right or wrong in yoga, as long as you are being safe and creating a practice that feels best for you.

A massive benefit of chair yoga is that doing these exercises on a regular basis will keep you safe on a regular basis. As we all know, with aging comes the risk of falls. According to the CDC, one in four seniors will experience a fall each year in the United States. This is often due to a decline in muscle mass, mobility, flexibility, balance, and a lack of physical activity. Fortunately, many of these concerns that come with aging can be mitigated by incorporating interventions such as chair yoga into our daily lives. Chair yoga helps reduce the risk of falls and injuries because it strengthens core muscles and improves proprioception. Our core muscles are activated during many chair yoga poses, which promotes stability and balance in the body. This also enhances proprioception as it improves body awareness.

Proprioception is a process that happens quickly within our brains; it is our body's ability to sense movement, spatial orientation, and position without relying on our vision. It describes where our body is with regard to our environment. Chair yoga optimizes this process by stimulating our sensory-motor pathways through poses and movements. Through consistent practice, this process becomes strengthened. Furthermore, the aspect of mindfulness encourages you to pay close attention to the sensations and movements within your body. This creates an increased sense of body positioning over time, leading to more stability. The movements in chair yoga are slow and controlled, which creates a strong connection between the mind and the body. It also involves movements that require you to shift your weight which challenges and strengthens your balance. All of these factors combined make chair yoga an optimal practice for naturally creating improved balance within your body.

Another exciting benefit of chair yoga is that it can assist in weight loss and management. As we get older, our metabolisms slow down, and maintaining a healthy weight can be challenging. Due to physical limitations, we become more susceptible to living a sedentary lifestyle. However, chair yoga helps us combat these issues and can actually promote weight loss. The gentle movements encourage circulation, increase metabolism, and support the body's natural detoxification pathways. Effective circulation within the body allows nutrients and oxygen to be delivered to the cells and waste products to be removed. This promotes a healthy metabolism which can contribute to weight loss. The movements in this practice stimulate the body's metabolism, which boosts the amount of calories your body burns. During the practice, you are burning calories which are essential in order to lose weight. The stretching encourages lymphatic flow throughout the body, which eliminates toxins and promotes detoxification. All of these benefits make chair yoga a valuable tool for weight loss or management and for promoting a healthy lifestyle overall.

If weight loss is something that you are aiming to achieve through this practice, it is also important to be mindful of nutrition in addition to implementing chair yoga into your life. Something that is interesting is that the awareness that is gained through your yoga practice can be applied to healthy eating patterns as well. As you continue to practice chair yoga and cultivate mindfulness, you will be much more in touch with your body and mind. Having this awareness will allow you to feel more connected to and aware of your hunger and fullness cues. This may sound too simple, but it is often overlooked. In general, it can be easy to overeat, which can lead to weight gain, especially when paired with a sedentary lifestyle. Whether it is due to stress or distractions, these things can make us mindlessly eat more calories than we actually need. Lowering our stress levels and cultivating awareness through practices like yoga allow us to combat mindless overeating. Essentially, being mindful and present while you eat can be highly beneficial to losing or maintaining weight. In addition, incorporating whole foods such as fruits, vegetables, grains, lean protein, and healthy fats is essential. Again, as you continue to practice yoga and become more mindful of how you feel within your body, you will naturally be more inclined to choose healthy foods that make you feel good. Through practicing chair yoga and eating healthily and mindfully, losing or maintaining your weight will become natural and effortless.

If you struggle with ailments such as arthritis, chronic pain, or overall stiffness, you could certainly benefit from practicing chair yoga. The stretches, gentle movements, and mindful relaxation techniques provide relief from discomfort. Stretching increases your range of motion and can reduce stiffness in your muscles and joints. The movements in yoga target specific muscle groups, which makes them stronger. Strengthening muscles, in turn, provides support around painful areas in the body. The aspect of mindfulness allows for a reduction in stress. Stress is known to exacerbate chronic pain, so decreasing your stress levels through this mindful practice can be beneficial. The breathing techniques incorporated into yoga promote relaxation and stress reduction as well, which leads to a decrease in pain perception. In addition, releasing endorphins that come with physical activity is key. Endorphins are natural pain-relieving chemicals found in our body and released during this practice. The holistic approach of yoga leads to an overall improvement in the mind and body.

The mind-body connection that is curated through chair yoga leads to stress reduction, improved mood, and mental clarity. Chair yoga activates the parasympathetic nervous system, also known as "rest and digest." This state is triggered by relaxation techniques, gentle movements, and breathing techniques that are incorporated into chair yoga. Activating the parasympathetic state leads to a decrease in heart rate, a decrease in blood pressure, the relaxation of smooth muscles, and improved respiratory function allowing for deeper breathing, optimal digestion, and the release of GABA. GABA is a neurochemical that promotes a calming effect. This neurochemical is associated with reduced anxiety and improved mood.

In addition, yoga supports the building of new neural pathways when practiced consistently, which can change the structure of the brain. This is often referred to as neuroplasticity, and it can lead to improved memory, increased attention, and an improved ability to learn and process information effectively. Studies even show that yoga could potentially be used as a tool to combat age-related neurodegenerative diseases like Alzheimer's. During the practice, you experience increased awareness and attention to the present moment. Focusing on movements, the breath, and bodily sensations cultivate a deep sense of presence. This leads to a calmer state of mind and can help you create a deeper understanding of your emotions, thoughts, and body.

Chair yoga is ideal for all older men and women because it is easily modifiable to meet your personal needs. Fitness facilities can be daunting and are not always accessible, which can be a barrier to exercising. Sometimes, physical limitations make it difficult to exercise there as well. It can also be expensive to join fitness centers which can be a barrier to exercising. We all have at least one sturdy chair in our home, so there's no barrier to initiating this practice. Practicing from the comfort of your own home is also ideal if you feel uncomfortable exercising in public. Regardless of how much space you have available to practice, you can easily practice chair yoga and experience the benefits. Another reason why it is ideal for all older men and women is because the risk of injury is low. As long as you do not push beyond your limits and follow the instructed poses properly, you will be able to safely practice chair yoga.

Now that we've discussed what chair yoga is and what the benefits of the practice are, we can dive into some of the dos and don'ts of chair yoga. When starting off with the do's, it is crucial to listen to your body during this practice. If something feels wrong or painful, stop the pose. It is essential to honor your limits and adjust the poses as needed in order to prevent discomfort or strain. You should also make sure to maintain proper body alignment while practicing. This means that you should engage your core muscles, keep your spine straight, and maintain good posture during the exercise. Another thing that you should do is warm up before getting started and cool down afterward. Preparing your body for movement is essential in order to prevent injury, and cooling down is crucial to encourage recovery and relaxation.

Furthermore, breathing deeply during the practice is beneficial. Using your breath to relax into the poses and breathing with the movements enhances the practice. And finally, using props and modifications as needed is critical. Blocks, cushions, or straps can be helpful to support your poses. Blocks are supportive devices that you can use to make poses more accessible. For instance, they can be used to support your feet during certain poses. Cushions can be placed behind your back or bottom to support you, provide comfort, and encourage proper alignment. Finally, straps can be used to help you stretch and increase your range of motion. For example, you can use a strap to encourage your arms into a shoulder stretch. In addition, modifying the poses to meet your personal abilities and needs will result in a safe and effective practice.

Let's take a look at some of the "don'ts" of chair yoga. First and foremost, do not neglect chair stability. Make sure that the chair you use is sturdy and secure for safety. Do not use a chair that is unstable, wobbly, or uncomfortable. There are a few things that you should look out for. Make sure to check your chair for any signs of damage, like loose screws or cracks. Also, make sure that the weight-bearing capacity of your chair is appropriate for your current weight. And finally, make sure that the feet of the chair have a non-slip surface or pad to prevent sliding during your practice. Do not force yourself into a position that feels uncomfortable or painful for you. As we mentioned before, modify or omit the poses that do not feel right for your body. Do not hold your breath during the practice. This can happen unconsciously sometimes when we are stressed or eager, so it is important to be mindful. Holding your breath can lead to tension within the body, so keeping a relaxed and steady breath during the practice is optimal. Do not move abruptly and quickly. Instead, move smoothly and mindfully when getting into or changing poses. Jerky movements can lead to joint or muscle strain, so it is best to be slow and gentle during your practice.

Chair yoga is a practice that should empower you to listen to the needs of your mind and body. We previously touched on the importance of honoring your specific needs and respecting your limitations, and this is essential to be kept in mind during the practice. Not only is this important for your physical safety, but for your mental health as well. Starting something new can be intimidating, so be gentle and patient with yourself. Chair yoga will be easy to understand and learn through this guide, but I still want to remind you that it is okay to stumble and make mistakes. There is no need to judge yourself throughout your practice, as you will improve as time goes on. You should be proud of yourself for choosing to participate in this practice and supporting your physical and mental well-being. Through consistency and repetition, you will become more familiar and comfortable with the various poses and stretches. Taking it one day at a time and giving yourself grace is a great way to approach your practice. Observing your thoughts and physical body through a non-judgmental lens is what yoga is all about.

In this chapter, we talked about how chair yoga came to be. We also discussed how it is accessible to pretty much anyone and how it is especially beneficial for seniors over 60 and individuals with physical limitations or injuries. We uncovered the abundance of mental and physical benefits that come with this practice. These benefits included a decreased risk for falls; improvements in flexibility, balance, and mobility; improved mood and mental clarity; a decrease in stress and an increase in relaxation; weight loss and weight management; pain relief from various chronic conditions; and more. We explored the importance of listening to your body, maintaining proper alignment, and taking safety measures during your practice. I want to emphasize that this practice can be adjusted as needed in order to meet your mental and physical needs. In the next chapter, we will dive into step-by-step instructions on how you can get started with your chair yoga practice.

CHAPTER 2:
GETTING STARTED WITH CHAIR YOGA

Now, we will be getting into more details about chair yoga and how you can actually begin your own practice. As we've mentioned many times, you are fully capable of incorporating chair yoga into your daily life and reaping the benefits of this practice. Even if you haven't exercised in years or have never tried any form of yoga, you will easily be able to learn and apply this practice to your life. When starting off, it is important to start slowly and to be patient with yourself. In order to build a consistent routine, making the practice a peaceful and enjoyable process is key. This is achieved through being non-judgemental with yourself and allowing room for error. This guide will make it very simple for you to begin practicing the poses, breathing techniques, and relaxation exercises, but remember to take things one step at a time. I'm sure you've heard the phrase, "Rome was not built in one day." Similarly, your yoga practice will not be perfect overnight. It will take consistency, repetition, and patience with yourself. As time goes on, the practice will become more natural to you. You will go from reading through this guide and possibly feeling uncertain to being a seasoned chair yogi. Everyone has to start somewhere! There is no better time to begin than right now.

The sooner you start and stay consistent, the sooner you will improve and reap the benefits of this practice. The more consistent you are, the more likely you are to experience the life-long benefits of this ancient healing practice.

Approaching this practice with an open mind will lead you to explore and discover your own unique potential for your physical and mental well-being. You may currently have some limitations when it comes to what you can achieve. Maybe there are thoughts that are lingering in the back of your mind that sound like "I'm too weak" or "I'm too old," and I want you to release these ideas. Instead of fueling these thoughts and holding yourself back, consider other affirmations that you can say to yourself when initiating this practice. For instance, "I am getting stronger each day through my practice" or "I do not allow my age to define me." While it may feel unnatural to say these things initially, it is important to nudge yourself with positive thoughts. As you continue to focus on what you can achieve and how you can grow, your mental and physical health will expand for the better. We often limit ourselves before we even begin to try, and that is no way to live life. So make sure that you are reminding yourself that you are fully capable of practicing chair yoga and experiencing the benefits that you'd love to experience. It is never too late to start something new; remember this! You are getting closer and closer to a healthier mind and body just by reading this guide alone. You are expanding your awareness and learning about a practice that could transform you in many different ways. As you start implementing chair yoga into your daily routine, you will slowly begin to feel the power of this transformative journey.

Now that we've addressed any limiting beliefs that you may have, we can get into the fundamentals of the actual practice of chair yoga. We will clearly explain the poses, breathing techniques, and relaxation exercises that are a part of this practice. By having a basic understanding of these three components, you will be able to begin your chair yoga journey with ease and confidence. The poses we will discuss are designed to be completed while sitting on a chair. However, there are certain poses in which you can stand up if that is something that you feel comfortable doing. This is fully up to your own physical needs, and it is important that you start with the easier poses initially. Breathing techniques are an essential aspect of chair yoga as they encourage stress reduction, relaxation, and an increase in mindfulness. These breathing techniques can be practiced anywhere while sitting in a chair. We will touch on breathing awareness exercises which will allow you to create a deeper sense of presence and a stronger connection between your mind and body. The relaxation techniques that we will uncover are intended to quiet your mind, release any tension throughout the body, and simply experience a deeply relaxed state. Through guided imagery, progressive muscle relaxation, and other exercises, you will be able to experience a deep sense of mental and physical relaxation with these techniques. As we mentioned, mindful movement, proper alignment, and breathing awareness are crucial aspects of this practice. Pay close attention to your body's signals and adjust any of these techniques as needed to meet your unique needs.

We will explain various chair yoga poses. If you'd like to try them all out, one at a time, feel free to get into it. In the following chapter, we will provide you with a guide that you can follow when trying out these poses (as well as the breathing and relaxation techniques). Let's dive into some of the yoga poses that you can begin to incorporate into your practice:

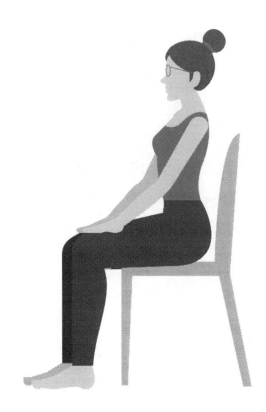

1. Seated Mountain Pose:

a. Sit tall on your chair with your feet planted flat on the ground, just about hip-width apart.

b. Put your hands on your thighs with your palms facing down.

c. Lengthen your spine through good posture (sitting up straight)

d. Relax your shoulders and elongate your neck, maintaining alignment with your spine

e. Take some deep breaths (inhaling deeply from your nose and exhaling through your nose)

f. Find stability in the pose, focus on your breath, and become aware of the present moment.

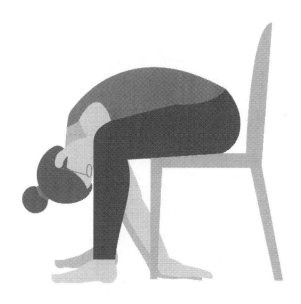

2. Seated Forward Fold:

a. Sit near the edge of the chair while keeping your feet flat on the floor.

b. Take an inhale through your nose, lift your chest up, and lengthen your spine.

c. Exhale through your nose while hinging forward from your hips, maintaining a flat back.

d. Let your hands reach toward your thighs, shins, or feet (whatever is most comfortable for you and your level of flexibility). If possible, put your hands on the floor (as shown in the image), but do not over-extend yourself and be very careful.

e. Allow your shoulders to relax and allow your head to gently drop downward.

f. Take some deep breaths and feel the stretch through the backside of your body (your legs and spine).

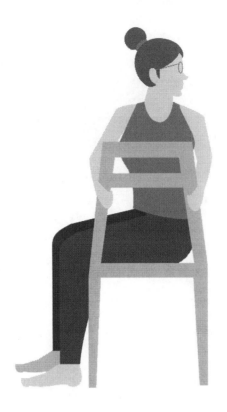

3. Seated Twist:

a. Take a seat sideways on your chair, keeping your right side closer to the backrest.

b. Inhale through your nose, lengthen through your spine, and put your left hand on the outer edge of your right thigh.

c. Exhale through your nose and twist your torso to the right gently. You can use your left hand to deepen the stretch as needed.

d. Ensure that your head is in alignment with your spine, or slightly look over your right shoulder to deepen the stretch.

e. Take deep breaths and feel the stretch; engage your core by flexing your abdominal muscles.

f. Repeat this exercise on the other side by switching the positioning of your legs and arms.

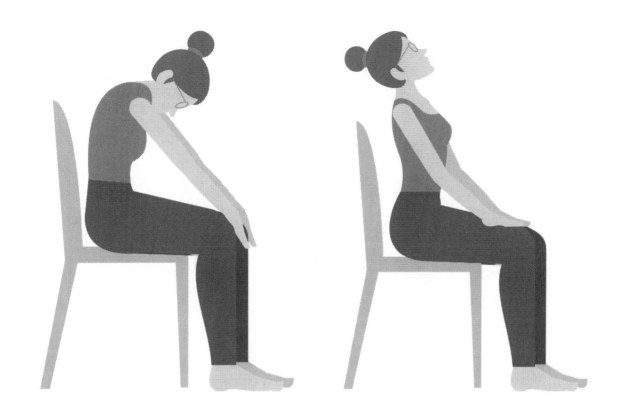

4. Seated Cat-Cow Stretch:

a. Begin by sitting tall on the chair, keeping your feet flat on the ground.

b. Put your hands on your thighs with your palms facing down.

c. Take an inhale and simultaneously arch your spine, lifting your chest forward (this is the Cow pose).

d. As you exhale, round your spine and slightly suck your stomach in, as if you are bringing your belly button inward towards your spine (this is the Cat pose).

e. Coordinate the Cow pose and Cat pose with your breath (inhaling during Cow and exhaling during Cat); smoothly slow between these two positions.

f. Feel the movement of your spin and the opening of your chest as you flow through the positions.

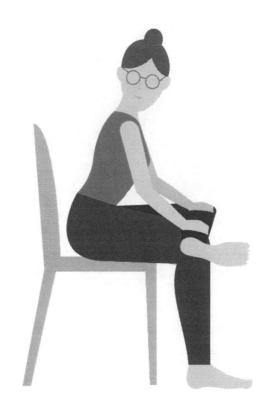

5. Seated Pigeon Pose:

a. Sit up tall on your chair and keep your feet flat on the floor.

b. Lift your right leg up and cross your ankle over your left thigh, let your right knee open up to the side. Keep your right foot flexed in order to protect your knee.

c. Ensure that your spine is long and then carefully hinge forward from your hips.

d. Put your hands on your right shin or carefully press on your right knee if you would like to deepen the stretch.

e. Breathe deeply through the stretch in your right hip and outer thigh.

f. Repeat this process on the other side, by crossing your left ankle over your right thigh and following the same steps.

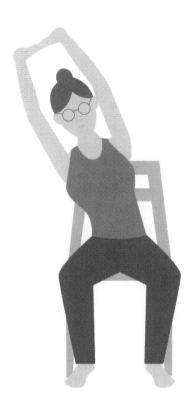

6. Seated Side Stretch:

a. Sit on the chair and put your feet flat on the floor, maintaining good posture.

b. Interlace your fingers and bring your arms overhead (extended).

c. Take an inhale and reach upward.

d. Exhale and lean to the ride side gently; you should feel a stretch along your left waist.

e. Ensure that your shoulders are relaxed during this stretch.

f. Inhale and come back to the center.

g. Repeat this on the left side and continue to alternate sides.

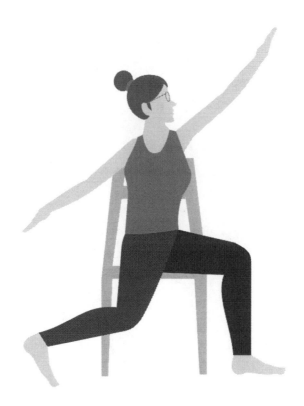

7. Seated Warrior I

a. Sit down on your chair and move closer to the front edge of your chair.

b. Slowly turn your body to the right side and move your bottom near the left edge of the chair in order to centralize yourself and create support for your right thigh (you are essentially turning sideways; you can use the back of your chair for support).

c. Keep your right hip on the chair and extend your left leg toward the floor, aligning the knee below the hip.

d. Press through the left foot and if you'd like to deepen the pose, extend your left leg back behind you and straighten it out as much as possible (based on your own flexibility and comfort).

e. Keep your arms at your hips or lengthen your body through your left arm.

f. Hold this pose for several deep breaths.

g. Repeat this on the other side.

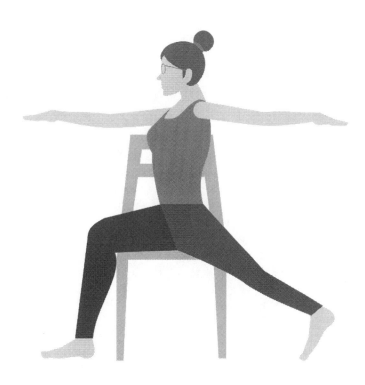

8. Seated Warrior II

a. Sit down on your chair and move closer toward the front of your chair.

b. Put your right leg out to the right side of your chair, angling your toes straight out (your foot should be perpendicular to the chair). Bend your knee on this side.

c. Step your left foot to the left side and position your foot parallel to your chair while keeping your left leg straight.

d. You can keep your hands on your hips or reach your arms out on either side, straight out from your shoulders. They should be parallel to the floor below you.

e. Move your shoulder blades away from your ears.

f. Rotate your ribcage to the left side until your chest faces the right side and gaze toward your right hand.

g. Repeat this pose on the other side, switching the legs.

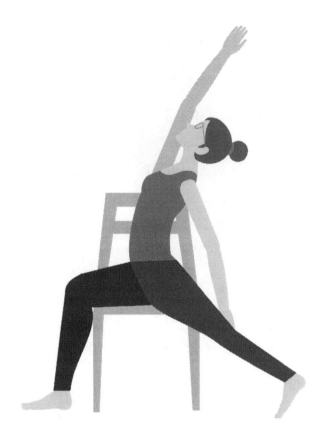

9. Chair Reverse Warrior

a. From the position you were in during Chair Warrior II, you can initiate this pose.

b. With your arms stretched out, inhale and slowly tilt your left arm down as your right arm goes up. You should feel a side stretch through your torso area.

c. Ensure that your neck is long and that your core muscles are engaged

d. Repeat this exercise on the other side.

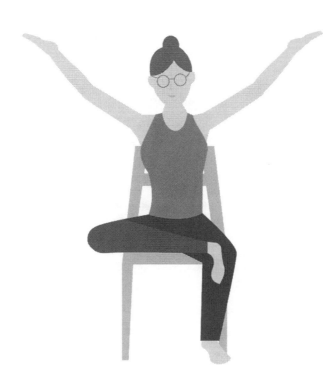

10. Seated Tree Pose

a. Sit on your chair and place your feet flat on the floor.

b. Place your left foot on the ground.

c. Lift your right foot and place it on top of your left thigh. If it is more comfortable for you, you could also just put the sole of your right foot against your inner left calf.

d. Find balance in this position and bring your hands to your heart center in a prayer pose. You can also raise your arms overhead like branches of a tree for this pose.

e. Take deep breaths and make sure to lengthen your spine and engage your core.

f. Hold this pose and breathe deeply. Repeat this on the other side, switching the positioning of your legs.

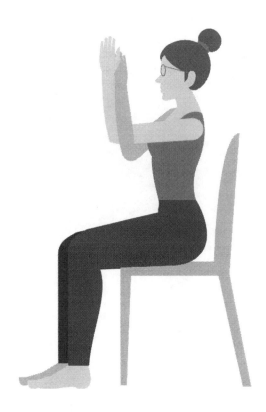

11. Seated Eagle Arms

a. Sit in your chair with your feet flat on the ground.

b. Extend your arms directly before you, keeping them at shoulder height.

c. First, cross your right arm over your left arm, and touch your palms together if it is possible (be gentle as always).

d. If you cannot touch your palms together, put the back of your right hand on top of your left palm.

e. Carefully lift your elbows; you should feel a soft stretch along your shoulders and upper back.

f. Take a few deep breaths as you hold this position.

g. Release the position and repeat the same stretch on the other side.

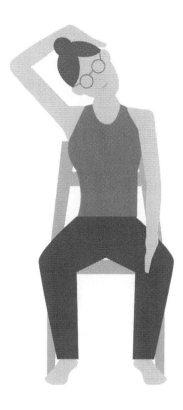

12. Seated Neck Stretch

a. Begin with your feet flat on the floor, sitting tall.

b. Drop your right ear onto your right shoulder while keeping your left shoulder nice and relaxed.

c. If you would like to deepen the stretch, use your right to lightly press the left side of your head.

d. Remain in this position for about 30 seconds to one minute while breathing deeply.

e. Release the position and move your head back to the center.

f. Repeat this same stretch on the opposite side.

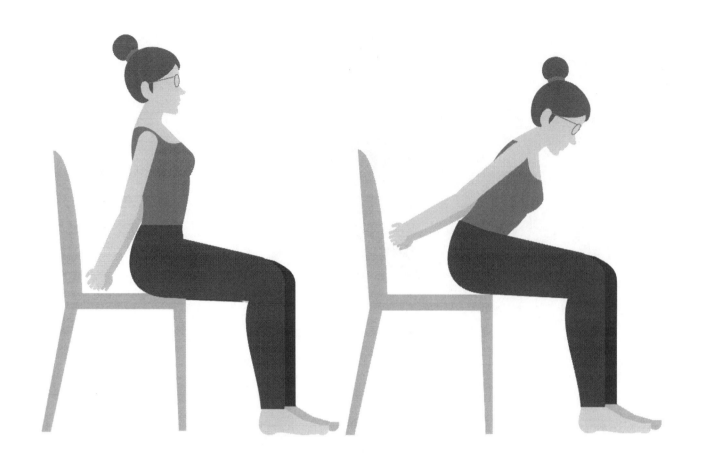

13. Seated Chest Opener

a. Take a seat closer to the front edge of your chair, keeping your feet flat on the ground.

b. Gently put your hands behind your back and interlace your fingers, keeping your palms facing inward.

c. Carefully squeeze your shoulder blades together and very gently lift your hands away from your lower back.

d. While you lift your hands in this position, let your chest open up and expand freely.

e. Breathe deeply in this position and feel the stretch in your chest and your shoulders.

f. Release this position by releasing the interlace of your fingers and bringing your hands back to rest in your lap.

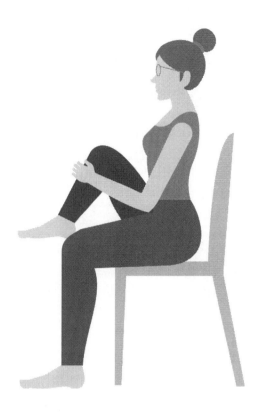

14. Seated Knee Lifts

a. Sit with your feet flat on the ground, hands resting comfortably on your thighs.

b. Start by slowly lifting your right knee up towards your chest, and keep your left foot flat on the floor.

c. As you are lifting your knee, hold onto your right thigh with your hands for extra support. If you are comfortable with doing so, lift your leg up closer to your chest.

d. Take a pause and feel the stretch going through your thigh and hip as you breathe.

e. Slowly and gently release your right foot back to the floor and take a pause.

f. Do the same stretch on the opposite side (your left leg).

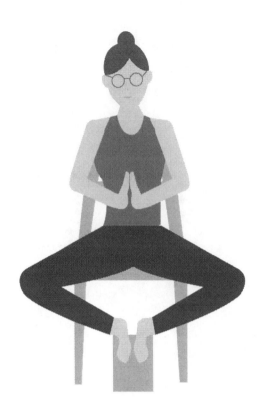

15. Seated Butterfly Stretch

a. Take a seat slightly closer toward the front of your seat, keeping your feet flat on the floor.

b. Optional: if you have a yoga block, you can place this under your feet, as you can see in the image.

c. Connect the soles of your feet together and allow your knees to slowly and gently open out to the sides.

d. Lightly press on your knees to deepen the stretch and sit tall.

e. If needed, hold on to your thighs for support. You can also bring your arms to a prayer position, connecting your palms together.

f. You should feel a stretch throughout your inner thighs and hips.

g. If you feel comfortable and feel like you can deepen the stretch, slightly lean forward (hinging from your hips). Ensure that your back is straight and take it slow.

h. Remain in this position while breathing deeply and then carefully release it. Bring your feet back, remaining flat on the floor.

Now that we've covered various poses that you can implement into your yoga practice, let us get into the breathing techniques. Your breath is extremely powerful, and it is something that is often overlooked. Breathing is our second nature and source of life, but how we breathe can impact us significantly. For instance, we can use our breath to calm us down and ground us. You may hold your breath or take rapid and shallow breaths when stressed. It is possible to gently get yourself out of that stressful state of mind by bringing awareness to your breath and slowing down your breathing. When we learn to slow our breath down, our mind will also slow down, putting us into a more calm headspace.

There are a few things to prepare for any breathing technique that you should keep in mind before beginning. First of all, find a comfortable and quiet place to begin this practice. You can do them on your yoga chair, with or without poses, or pretty much anywhere. Even if you are overwhelmed in public and feel as though you need to calm down, many breathing techniques can be done at any time. After trying out the ones that we will cover below, you can see which ones you feel would be appropriate to utilize when in public or out and about. It is best to be in a seated position with your spine straight, with your body relaxed, and your feet planted onto the ground. Your hands can rest in the position that feels most natural to you. If you would like, you can set an intention for this breathing practice. Maybe you'd like to decrease your stress, become more relaxed, increase your focus, or focus on any other intention. The practice is uniquely yours, so it is fully up to you. Before diving into the breathing exercises themselves, it is important to begin by focusing on your breath and starting with a few deep breaths to ground yourself. Connecting to your breath initially makes transitioning into specific exercises more seamless. Make sure to follow the guidelines and be mindful during this practice. If you feel uncomfortable, lightheaded, or dizzy, pause your practice and return to your normal breathing pattern. Stay present, observe your breath and the sensations within your body, and sink into the relaxing effects of these exercises.

Let's get into some breathing exercises you can begin to incorporate into your yoga practice. You can combine these with the poses or practice them alone:

1. Deep Belly Breathing

a. While sitting on your chair, place your hands on your belly.
b. Breathe deeply and slowly through your nose; you should feel your belly rise.
c. Take a slow exhale through your mouth as your belly falls inward.
d. Repeat this exercise for multiple breaths.

2. The 4-7-8 Breath

a. Take a complete exhale and make an audible sigh as you do so.
b. Close your mouth and take an inhale from your nose, counting to four.
c. Pause and hold your breath; count to seven.
d. Take an exhale through your mouth while counting to eight.
e. Repeat this a few times; this is especially great to do if you feel anxious in public settings.

3. Counted Breaths

a. Take a deep inhale through your nose and count to four, filling your lungs.
b. Exhale through your mouth while counting to six, completely releasing the breath.
c. Take a brief pause at the end of your exhale.

d. Repeat this multiple times, maintaining a relaxed state.

4. Alternate Nostril Breathing:

a. Gently put your right thumb over the side of your right nostril to close it off.

b. Take a deep inhale through your left nostril.

c. Once you have fully inhaled, use the ring finger of that same hand to close your left nostril and simultaneously release the right thumb so that your right nostril is open.

d. Full exhale through your right nostril.

e. Take a deep inhale through your right nostril and cover it with your thumb to close the nostril. Then exhale from the left nostril.

f. Alternate between the left and right nostrils, covering and uncovering them intermittently as described.

5. Three-Part Breath:

a. Take a deep inhale and fill your entire belly, ribcage, and chest with the air.

b. Slowly exhale and release the air from your chest, ribcage, and belly (reversing the flow)

c. Repeat this several times and focus on smoothly transitioning between the sections.

6. Cooling Breath:

a. Start by curling your tongue. Slowly inhale through it, feeling the cool air enter your mouth.

b. Exhale through your nose while closing your mouth. Touch the tip of your tongue to the roof of your mouth.

c. If you cannot curl your tongue, then purse your lips (create a rounded shape by bringing your lips together) and inhale through your mouth.

d. Repeat this technique for several breaths.

7. Lion's Breath:

a. Sit with good posture and put your hands on your knees.

b. Take a deep inhale through your nose.

c. Exhale through your mouth and simultaneously stick your tongue out straight, open your eyes wide, and make a "ha" sound. Take a deep breath through your nose. As you exhale through your mouth, stick out your tongue, widen your eyes, and forcefully let out a "ha" sound.

d. Repeat this breath multiple times and feel the release of tension.

8. Humming Bee Breath:

a. Sit comfortably and close your eyes gently.

b. Put your index fingers on the cartilage of your ears and close your eyes; take a deep inhale through your nose.

c. As you exhale, make a humming sound and feel the vibration of the hum in your body.

d. Do this for a few rounds.

9. Equal Breathing (Box Breathing):

a. Start by taking an inhale through your nose and count to four.

b. Hold your breath and count to four.

c. Exhale your breath and count to four.

d. Then again, hold your breath for a count of four.

e. Repeat this process for several rounds and watch as your mind and body calm down.

10. Diaphragmatic Breath:

a. Put one hand on your chest and then place your other hand on your belly.

b. As you take a slow and deep, inhale through your nose, feel your belly rise with your hand.

c. As you slowly exhale through your mouth, feel your belly fall with your hand as the breath leaves your body.

d. Breathe deeply into your diaphragm (the muscle below your heart and lunges). Expand your belly while inhaling and contract it as you exhale.

e. Do these diaphragmatic breaths for multiple rounds.

Now that we have covered the various poses and breathing exercises, we can get into some relaxation techniques you can implement. These techniques allow you to enter a more calm state, mentally and physically. When stressed, we often feel as though our thoughts are running wild and we may even feel tension throughout our bodies. In order to return to a more relaxed state, we can use these interventions to guide us back to a place of peace and calmness. You can practice these exercises from your yoga chair, couch, bed, or any location. Some of these techniques will suggest that you lie down for the best results. These exercises are amazing for reducing stress, enhancing your mind-body connection, physical relaxation and comfort, and even improving your sleep quality. Let's cover some relaxation exercises that you can start to incorporate into your routine:

1. Progressive Muscle Relaxation

a. Take a seat and gently close your eyes.

b. Begin by taking a few deep breaths and relaxing into your body.

c. Begin by tensing the muscles within your feet and toes, holding for a few seconds.

d. Release this tension and feel the relaxation of doing so.

e. Moving upward to your legs, tense the calve muscles, hold for a few seconds, and release.

f. Move your attention upward, repeating the same action of tensing, holding, and releasing. Move up to your thighs, then bottom and pelvic area, abdomen, hands and arms, shoulders, neck, and face.

g. As you release the tension, release any tightness that may be found in any area of your body. Allow the relaxation to overcome you.

h. Repeat this if you still feel any areas of tension.

2. Guided Visualization

a. Sit or lie down comfortably, and gently close your eyes.

b. Take a few deep breaths and release any tension in your body.

c. Begin by visualizing yourself in a location that is peaceful to you. This may be the beach, a quiet forest, or up in the mountains. It can be any location that feels beautiful and calming to you.

d. Envision the sensations that you would experience while being in this location. Imagine the smells, the sounds, and the textures of the surroundings in your chosen setting.

e. Take a few minutes to completely immerse yourself in this mental image. Allow yourself to feel the peace and relaxation of mentally being in this area.

3. Guided Deep Relaxation (Yoga Nidra)

a. We will begin by lying on our backs for this position; in bed, on a mat, or anywhere that is comfortable for you.

b. Lie with your palms facing the sky and your legs gently spread out.

c. Initially, focus on your right foot and let your awareness remain there for a few seconds. Slowly relax your right foot and divert your attention to your right knee, the right thigh, and the right hip.

d. After drawing attention to each part of the right leg, bring your awareness to your entire leg and allow it to fully relax. Take a deep inhale and exhale.

e. Repeat this same process with your left foot, bringing your awareness upwards and then to the left leg.

f. Continue this process by bringing your awareness to each part of your body and then relaxing them. Go upwards to your pelvic and bottom area, your abdomen, chest, back, right arm and shoulder, left arm and shoulder, neck area, and head area.

g. Breathe deeply throughout the process and become aware of your entire body.

h. Once you have gone through each body part, relax here for a little bit.

i. After a few minutes, bring your awareness back to the present moment. Takes some deep breaths and gently open your eyes when you're ready.

4. Body Scan Meditation

a. Begin in a sitting position or lying down.

b. Gently close your eyes and take some deep breaths to settle into your body.

c. Begin by bringing awareness to the top of your head and slowly go down through your body.

d. Scan each body part for any feelings of tension. Allow any areas of tension to slowly soften as you take a deep breath; let the muscles soften.

e. Keep scanning down through your neck, shoulders, arms, chest, abdomen, hips, legs, and feet.

f. Maintain presence and feel the sensations in each part of your body; relax and let go.

g. Do not rush yourself through this process, going from head to toe.

h. Once you've reached the end of your body scan, take some time to bask in the relaxed state of your body.

i. Slowly open your eyes and return to the present when you are ready.

5. Breath Counting

a. Begin by sitting comfortably (this can be done in any position) and close your eyes.

b. Gently bring your attention to your breath. Do not try to change the pattern. Simply observe it.

c. When you inhale, count "one." When you exhale, count "two." When you inhale again, count "three." When you exhale, count "four."

d. Repeat this pattern until you reach ten. Once you do, you can start again from one.

e. If you get distracted or lose count, return your focus to your breath and start from the beginning.

f. Repeat this as needed in order to calm down or create focus within your mind.

In this chapter, we covered a variety of poses, breathing exercises, and relaxation techniques that you can begin to try out. Whether you'd like to start with poses alone, breathing exercises alone, relaxation techniques alone, or a combination of all of them is up to you. These gentle and accessible techniques will be an amazing addition to your daily or weekly routine. As you now know, doing chair yoga is one of the best things that you can do for your physical and mental health. Remember not to overwhelm yourself as you learn about the stretches and breathwork. Start slowly and build on your practice as you become more comfortable with the techniques. In the next chapter, we will talk about how you can gradually incorporate these techniques into your practice. We will get into how you can embrace your journey and truly appreciate the process of learning chair yoga with curiosity and enthusiasm.

CHAPTER 3:

CHAIR YOGA PROGRAM
FOR BEGINNERS.

If you feel overwhelmed by the amount of information you have just learned, I want to remind you that taking this practice one step at a time is important. It is best to begin with poses and breathing techniques that are more simple and to start incorporating the more complex ones slowly. We will elaborate on that throughout this chapter. Regardless of your fitness level, body type, or age, you will be able to implement this practice into your life successfully. Any pose can be modified to lessen or deepen the stretch that is taking place. Any breathing or relaxation techniques that you don't quite enjoy do not have to be a part of your routine. The beauty of this practice is that it is uniquely yours. In addition, to incorporate any practice into your life, gradually introducing it into your daily routine is best. Setting aside a specific time that you would like to practice chair yoga each day will help you stay consistent. Maybe it will be a part of your morning routine or your nightly routine.

If you start off doing many different poses on your first day for a long time, you may overwhelm yourself. Being gentle and slowly getting acquainted with the practice will make it easier for you to continue doing it and actually enjoy it. With consistency, you will begin to experience an increase in your flexibility, balance, and strength, as well as improvements in your overall physical and mental well-being. You could begin by testing out a few poses and breathing techniques and then choosing the ones that feel best for your specific needs. Starting off with just a few minutes a day and then building up to 10-minute periods or more will allow you to sustain this practice long-term. The time commitment is minimal, which makes this a very doable practice.

In this next section, we will provide a progressive chair yoga program that gives you some structure for beginning this practice. Feel free to do so if you want to move at a slower or faster pace. This is intended to be a guide that can be followed at your own pace and modified as needed. So that you don't have to flip back and forth between pages, we have included the description of each stretch and breathing/relaxation technique for each phase. Each phase can be practiced anywhere from a day to a week before moving on to the next phase.

Phase 1: The initial phase is intended to get you acquainted with the foundation of your chair yoga practice. You can set aside a few minutes to try out this pose and the breathing/relaxation techniques. If you feel like doing one pose is too simple, you can always add more poses that we mentioned earlier to create a flow (we will get into what a flow is during phase 5). These poses, breathing, and relaxation techniques are the most simple and foundational. We will build on these skills throughout the next few phases. You can move quicker or slower, depending on your comfort level.

- **Pose**: Seated Mountain Pose

    o Sit tall on your chair with your feet planted flat on the ground, just about hip-width apart.

    o Put your hands on your thighs with your palms facing down.

- o Lengthen your spine through good posture (sitting up straight)
- o Relax your shoulders and elongate your neck, maintaining alignment with your spine
- o Take some deep breaths (inhaling deeply from your nose and exhaling through your nose)
- o Find stability in the pose, focus on your breath, and become aware of the present moment.

- **Breathing Technique:** Deep Belly Breathing

  - o While sitting on your chair, put your hands on your belly.
  - o Slowly breathe deeply through your nose; you should feel your belly rise while doing so.
  - o Take a slow exhale through your mouth, feeling your belly fall inward.
  - o Repeat this exercise for multiple breaths.

- **Relaxation Technique:** Progressive Muscle Relaxation

  - o Take a seat and gently close your eyes.
  - o Begin by taking a few deep breaths and relaxing into your body.
  - o Begin by tensing the muscles within your feet and toes, holding for a few seconds.
  - o Release this tension and feel the relaxation of doing so.
  - o Moving upward to your legs, tense the calve muscles, hold for a few seconds, and release.
  - o Move your attention upward, repeating the same action of tensing, holding, and releasing. Move up to your thighs, then bottom and pelvic area, abdomen, hands and arms, shoulders, neck, and face.
  - o As you release the tension, release any tightness that may be found in any area of your body. Allow the relaxation to overcome you.

o   Repeat this if you still feel any areas of tension.

Phase 2: The poses in this phase are still very beginner friendly, but they involve a few more steps than the previous techniques that we touched on. You can now add this pose to your practice and slowly build it up in your regimen. The breathing techniques can be used at various times throughout your day or during the stretches as well. The relaxation technique, guided visualization, can be used during your practice or specifically for times of stress. It is important to practice this technique during a time when you can close your eyes and be fully immersed in the present moment.

- **Pose:** Seated Forward Fold

  o   Sit closer to the chair's edge while keeping your feet flat on the floor.
  o   Take an inhale through your nose, lift ur chest up, and lengthen your spine.
  o   Exhale through your nose while hinging forward from your hips, maintaining a flat back.
  o   Let your hands reach toward your thighs, shins, or feet (whatever is most comfortable for you and your level of flexibility).
  o   Allow your shoulders to relax and allow your head to gently drop downward.
  o   Take some deep breaths and feel the stretch through the backside of your body (your legs and spine).

- **Breathing Technique:** Three-Part Breath

  o   Take a deep inhale and fill your entire belly, ribcage, and chest with the air.

- o Slowly exhale and release the air from your chest, ribcage, and belly (reversing the flow)
- o Repeat this a couple of times and focus on smoothly transitioning between the sections.

- **Relaxation Technique:** Guided Visualization

  - o Sit or lie down comfortably, and gently close your eyes.
  - o Take a few deep breaths and release any tension in your body.
  - o Begin by visualizing yourself in a location that is peaceful to you. This may be the beach, a quiet forest, or up in the mountains. It can be any location that feels beautiful and calming to you.
  - o Envision the sensations that you would experience while being in this location. Imagine the smells, the sounds, and the textures of the surroundings in the setting you chose.
  - o Take a few minutes to completely immerse yourself in this mental image. Allow yourself to feel the peace and relaxation of mentally being in this area.

Phase 3: Now that you have mastered the first two phases and you have built a foundation for simple poses and breathing/relaxation techniques, we can move on to ones that are slightly more complex. These poses have a few more steps involved. There is also another pose added to this phase that may be slightly more challenging that you can try out. You can begin with the first pose and if it feels simple, feel free to try out the challenging pose as well. The breathing technique can be used while on the chair but may be hard to do simultaneously with poses (it involves using your hand). The relaxation technique of body scanning is great for calming down during the day or to wind down before bedtime. Sometimes we do not even realize our bodies are tense, so this technique is amazing for releasing any unknown tension.

- **Pose:** Seated Cat-Cow Pose

  - Begin by sitting tall on the chair, keeping your feet flat on the ground.
  - Put your hands on your thighs with your palms facing down.
  - Take an inhale and simultaneously arch your spine, lifting your chest forward (this is the Cow pose).
  - As you exhale, round your spine and bring your belly button towards your spine (this is the Cat pose).
  - Coordinate the Cow pose and Cat pose with your breath (inhaling during Cow and exhaling during Cat); smoothly slow between these two positions.
  - Feel the movement of your spin and the opening of your chest as you flow through the positions.

- **Challenging Pose:** Seated Twist

  - Take a seat sideways on your chair, keeping your right side closer to the backrest.
  - Inhale through your nose, lengthen through your spine, and put your left hand on the outer edge of your right thigh.
  - Exhale through your nose and twist your torso to the right gently. You can use your left hand to deepen the stretch as needed.
  - Ensure that your head is in alignment with your spine or slightly look over your right shoulder to deepen the stretch.
  - Take deep breaths and feel the stretch. Engage your core by flexing your abdominal muscles.
  - Repeat this exercise on the other side by switching the positioning of your legs and arms.

- **Breathing Technique:** Alternate Nostril Breathing

  o Gently put your right thumb over the side of your right nostril to close it off.

  o Take a deep inhale through your left nostril.

  o Once you have fully inhaled, use the ring finger of that same hand to close your left nostril and simultaneously release the right thumb so that your right nostril is open.

  o Full exhale through your right nostril.

  o Take a deep inhale through your right nostril and cover it with your thumb to close the nostril. Then exhale from the left nostril.

  o Alternate between the left and right nostrils, covering them and uncovering them intermittently as described.

- **Relaxation Technique:** Body Scan Meditation

  o Begin in a sitting position or lying down.

  o Gently close your eyes and take some deep breaths to settle into your body.

  o Begin by bringing awareness to the top of your head and slowly go down through your body.

  o Scan each body part for any feelings of tension. Allow any areas of tension to slowly soften as you take a deep breath; let the muscles soften.

  o Keep scanning down through your neck, shoulders, arms, chest, abdomen, hips, legs, and feet.

  o Maintain presence and feel the sensations in each part of your body; relax and let go.

  o Do not rush yourself through this process, going from head to toe.

  o Once you've reached the end of your body scan, take some time to bask in the relaxed state of your body.

o Slowly open your eyes and return to the present when you are ready.

Phase 4: These next few poses may seem a bit more challenging. There are more movements that need to be done in order to achieve the stretch, but it is still very achievable regardless of your limitations. Make sure to be gentle and slow; start off with the first pose, and then move on to trying out the more challenging pose. If you are more of a visual learner, we have attached photos in chapter two, where we explained these poses. There are also many Youtube videos that show you how to do these poses as well. The breathing technique that we will touch on is very simple and can be done anywhere. It is a great way to calm down by extending your exhale. The 4-7-8 technique is amazing to incorporate during stressful times or during your yoga practice. The relaxation technique is also quite simple and can be done wherever you are.

- **Pose:** Seated Warrior I

    o Sit down on your chair and move closer to the front edge of your chair.
    o Slowly turn your body to the right side and move your bottom near the left edge of the chair in order to centralize yourself and create support for your right thigh (you are essentially turning sideways; you can use the back of your chair for support).
    o Keep your right hip on the chair and extend your left leg toward the floor, aligning the knee below the hip.
    o Press through the left foot and if you'd like to deepen the pose, extend your left leg back behind you and straighten it out as much as possible (based on your own flexibility and comfort).
    o Keep your arms at your hips or lengthen your body through your left arm.
    o Hold this pose for several deep breaths.

- o Repeat this on the other side.

- **Challenging Pose:** Seated Tree Pose

  - o Sit on your chair with your feet flat on the floor.
  - o Place your left foot on the ground.
  - o Lift your right foot and put the sole against your inner left calf or left inner thigh.
  - o Find balance in this position and bring your hands to your heart center in a prayer pose. You can also raise your arms overhead like branches of a tree for this pose.
  - o Take deep breaths and make sure to lengthen your spine and engage your core.
  - o Hold this pose and breathe deeply. Repeat this on the other side, switching the positioning of your legs.

- **Breathing Technique: The** 4-7-8 Breath

  - o Take a complete exhale and make an audible sigh as you do so.
  - o Close your mouth and take an inhale from your nose as you count to four.
  - o Pause here and hold your breath while counting to seven.
  - o Take an exhale through your mouth while counting to eight.
  - o Repeat this a few times; this is especially great to do if you feel anxious in public settings.

- **Relaxation Technique:** Breath Counting

  - o Begin by sitting comfortably (this can be done in any position) and close your eyes.

- Gently bring your attention to your breath. Do not try to change the pattern. Simply observe it.
- When you inhale, count "one." When you exhale, count "two." When you inhale again, count "three." When you exhale, count "four."
- Repeat this pattern until you reach ten. Once you do, you can start again from one.
- If you get distracted or lose count, return your focus to your breath and start from the beginning.
- Repeat this as needed in order to calm down or create focus within your mind.

Phase 5: You have mastered multiple poses, so now, we can begin to create a flow sequence. A flow sequence is a series of poses that are linked together, one pose flowing into the next. The flow's speed, complexity, and intensity are fully up to you and your personal needs. Begin by trying out the poses independently, then combine the two into one sequence. As you get more comfortable doing the two poses back to back, you can combine more poses that you have practiced into your flow. You can begin by trying either one of the two flow sequence ideas. If you feel ready, you can combine them as well. Feel free to be creative and combine different poses that you enjoy practicing. We will touch on another breathing technique that can be done at any time. You can use box breathing to calm down during times of anxiety or stress, or you can use it during your yoga practice. The relaxation technique we will discuss encourages your mind and body to relax deeply. It is great for regulating your nervous system and helps promote deep sleep.

- **Flow Sequence 1:** Seated Side Stretch to a Seated Twist

  - Seated Side Stretch:

- Sit on the chair, keeping your feet flat on the floor with good posture.
- Interlace your fingers and bring your arms overhead (extended).
- Take an inhale and reach upward.
- Exhale and lean to the ride side gently; you should feel a stretch along your left waist.
- Ensure that your shoulders are relaxed during this stretch.
- Inhale and come back to the center.
- Repeat this on the left side and continue to alternate sides.

- (2) Seated Twist:

  - Take a seat sideways on your chair, keeping your right side closer to the backrest.
  - Inhale through your nose, lengthen through your spine, and put your left hand on the outer edge of your right thigh.
  - Exhale through your nose and twist your torso to the right gently. You can use your left hand to deepen the stretch as needed.
  - Ensure that your head is in alignment with your spine or slightly look over your right shoulder to deepen the stretch.
  - Take deep breaths and feel the stretch. Engage your core by flexing your abdominal muscles.
  - Repeat this exercise on the other side by switching the positioning of your legs and arms.

- **Flow Sequence 2**: Seated Cat-Cow to Seated Forward Fold

  - Seated Cat-Cow Stretch:

    - Begin by sitting tall on the chair, keeping your feet flat on the ground.
    - Put your hands on your thighs with your palms facing down.

- Take an inhale and simultaneously arch your spine, lifting your chest forward (this is the Cow pose).

- As you exhale, round your spine and slightly suck your stomach in, as if you are bringing your belly button inward towards your spine (this is the Cat pose).

- Coordinate the Cow pose and Cat pose with your breath (inhaling during Cow and exhaling during Cat); smoothly slow between these two positions.

- Feel the movement of your spin and the opening of your chest as you flow through the positions.

- (2) Seated Forward Fold

  - Sit near the chair's edge while keeping your feet flat on the floor.

  - Take an inhale through your nose, lift your chest up, and lengthen your spine.

  - Exhale through your nose while hinging forward from your hips, maintaining a flat back.

  - Let your hands reach toward your thighs, shins, or feet (whatever is most comfortable for you and your level of flexibility).

  - Allow your shoulders to relax and allow your head to drop downward gently.

  - Take some deep breaths and feel the stretch through the backside of your body (your legs and spine).

- **Breathing Technique:** Box Breathing

  - Start by taking an inhale through your nose and count to four.
  - Hold your breath and count to four.
  - Exhale your breath and count to four.

- o Then again, hold your breath for a count of four.

- o Repeat this process for several rounds and watch as your mind and body calm down.

- **Relaxation Technique:** Yoga Nidra

  - o You will begin by lying on your back for this position; in bed, on a mat, or anywhere comfortable for you.

  - o Lie with your palms facing the sky and your legs gently spread out.

  - o Focus on your right foot and let your awareness remain there for a few seconds. Slowly relax your right foot and divert your attention to your right knee, then the right thigh, and the right hip.

  - o After drawing attention to each part of the right leg, bring your awareness to your entire leg and allow it to relax fully. Take a deep inhale and exhale.

  - o Repeat this process with your left foot, bringing your awareness upwards and then to the left leg.

  - o Continue this process by bringing your awareness to each part of your body and then relaxing them. Go upwards to your pelvic and bottom area, your abdomen, chest, back, right arm and shoulder, left arm and shoulder, neck area, and head area.

  - o Breathe deeply throughout the process and become aware of your entire body.

  - o Once you have gone through each body part, relax here for a little bit.

  - o After a few minutes have passed, bring your awareness back to the present moment. Takes some deep breaths and gently open your eyes when you're ready.

In this chapter, we covered various poses, breathing techniques, and relaxation techniques you can utilize. Relaxation techniques can be used regularly in order to create stability within your mind. You may test out the various techniques and use the ones that make you feel the best. You can start your morning off with a relaxation technique to enter the day with a clear head. You can also end your day with a relaxation technique to clear your mind before going to bed, making it easier to fall asleep. The poses we touched on can be combined to create a simple flow. Breathing techniques such as box breathing and the 4-7-8 technique can be done as you perform the poses. The next chapter will explore more complex poses and yoga flows.

CHAPTER 4:

ADVANCED CHAIR
YOGA PROGRAM.

Now that you have tried out various foundational poses, stretches, and breathing techniques, we can move on to some more advanced practices. We briefly touched on the idea of yoga flows in the previous chapter and will build on this. We initially combined two poses into a flow, but we will be adding different poses into one sequence now. We will also give more details on how you can use breathwork throughout your practice. These facets will allow you to create a more extended yoga flow rather than just trying out a few poses here and there. Practicing about 10 minutes of chair yoga a day or more is optimal for experiencing long-term benefits. However, you can do this practice even longer if you are comfortable and ready. You can slowly begin to try out more challenging poses as you become more comfortable with the basic ones. We will also give you some examples of flow sequences that you can utilize alone or in combination with others to make up 10 minutes of yoga practice. Starting off with just a few minutes a day and then gradually building up the length of your routine is an excellent way to approach your journey.

Some foundational poses we touched on in the previous chapter include the seated mountain pose, the seated forward fold, the seated cat-cow pose, the seated twist, the seated warrior I, the seated tree pose, and the seated side stretch. We have also created flow sequences during the final phases. We will be adding more mini-flow lines throughout these phases to get you acquainted with the more challenging poses. If doing them back-to-back feels too difficult initially, feel free to do one at a time. In these next phases, we will also begin with a few foundational poses that we did not specifically touch on during the phases you went through in the previous chapter. These simple poses can be a part of your warm-up and are best paired with some of the breathing techniques we have described. In addition, we will incorporate the remaining breathing techniques that you can try out during each phase. We have fully covered the relaxation techniques, so feel free to use them as needed. As we mentioned previously, each step can be practiced anywhere from a day to a week, depending on fast or slow you'd like to move through.

Phase 1: In this phase, we will touch on some of the simple poses that we did not specifically mention in Phase 1 of the previous chapter. This phase is intended to be more of a warm-up so that we can slowly move into the more complex movements. At this point, you have tried out many different poses and simple yoga flows. In this chapter, each phase will have at least two poses (one regular pose and one challenging pose) to try out or a flow sequence. In addition, the breathing technique is added for you to test out at any time. The counting technique is a great one to incorporate while you do the poses because it keeps you in the present moment. It's easy for our thoughts to wander as we stretch, so focusing on counting our breaths can be helpful to slow down our thoughts.

- **Pose:** Seated Neck Stretch

    o Begin with your feet flat on the floor, sitting tall.

    o Drop your right ear onto your right shoulder while keeping your left shoulder nice and relaxed.

    o If you would like to deepen the stretch, use your right to press the left side of your head lightly.

    o Remain in this position for about 30 seconds to one minute while breathing deeply.

    o Release the position and move your head back to the center.

    o Repeat this same stretch on the opposite side.

- **Challenging Pose:** Seated Chest Opener

    o Take a seat closer to the front edge of your chair, keeping your feet flat on the ground.

    o Gently put your hands behind your back and interlace your fingers, keeping your palms facing inward.

    o Carefully squeeze your shoulder blades together and very gently lift your hands away from your lower back.

    o Let your chest open up and expand freely while you lift your hands in this position.

    o Breathe deeply in this position and feel the stretch in your chest and your shoulders.

    o Release this position by releasing the interlace of your fingers and bringing your hands back to rest in your lap.

- **Breathing technique:** Counted Breaths

    o Take a deep inhale through your nose and count to four, filling your lungs.

- Exhale through your mouth while counting to six, completely releasing the breath.
- Take a brief pause at the end of your exhale.
- Repeat this multiple times, maintaining a relaxed state.

Phase 2: The poses in this portion are slightly more advanced and require more steps than the previous ones. However, they are fully achievable. We touched on seated warrior I in the last chapter, and now we are getting into seated warrior II and reverse warrior. These poses can be combined to create a mini-flow sequence, which we have included below. The breathing exercise included in this phase helps calm yourself down and regulate your nervous system. It is great to do this breath during times of anxiety or discomfort.

- **Flow Sequence:** Seated Warrior II to Chair Reverse Warrior

  - Seated Warrior II

    - Sit down on your chair and move closer toward the front of your chair.
    - Put your right leg out to the right side of your chair, angling your toes straight out (your foot should be perpendicular to the chair). Bend your knee on this side.
    - Step your left foot to the left side and position your foot parallel to your chair while keeping your left leg straight.
    - You can keep your hands on your hips or reach your arms out on either side, straight out from your shoulders. They should be parallel to the floor below you.
    - Move your shoulder blades away from your ears.
    - Rotate your ribcage to the left side until your chest faces the right side, and gaze toward your right hand.

- o (2) Chair Reverse Warrior

  - From the position you were in during Chair Warrior II, you can initiate this pose.

  - With your arms stretched out, inhale and slowly tilt your left arm down as your right arm goes up. You should feel a side stretch through your torso area.

  - Ensure that your neck is long and that your core muscles are engaged.

Repeat this flow on the other side, starting from the beginning

- **Breathing Technique:** Cooling Breath

  - o Start by curling your tongue. Slowly inhale through it, feeling the cool air enter your mouth.

  - o Exhale through your nose while closing your mouth. Touch the tip of your tongue to the roof of your mouth.

  - o If you cannot curl your tongue, then purse your lips (create a rounded shape by bringing your lips together) and inhale through your mouth.

  - o Repeat this technique for several breaths.

Phase 3: We are now touching on poses focusing on lower body strength. These poses flow nicely into one another and can be added to a longer sequence. It is important to note that these poses can be modified to meet your level of flexibility. If you feel uncomfortable performing any poses, you may skip them altogether. When lifting your knee up, be very gentle and move slowly. Once you meet mild resistance, allow yourself to feel the stretch, and do not over-exert yourself. The breathing technique of diaphragmatic breaths can be performed before or after your sequence of poses or at any time.

- **Flow Sequence:** Seated Pigeon to Seated Knee Lift

  o Seated Pigeon Pose

    - Sit up tall on your chair and keep your feet flat on the floor.
    - Lift your right leg up, cross your ankle over your left thigh, and let your right knee open to the side. Keep your right foot flexed in order to protect your knee.
    - Ensure that your spine is long, and then carefully hinge forward from your hips.
    - Put your hands on your right shin or carefully press on your right knee if you would like to deepen the stretch.
    - Breathe deeply through the stretch in your right hip and outer thigh.
    - Repeat this process on the other side by crossing your left ankle over your right thigh and following the same steps.

  o (2) Seated Knee Lift

    - Sit with your feet flat on the ground, hands resting comfortably on your thighs.
    - Start by slowly lifting your right knee up towards your chest, and keep your left foot flat on the floor.
    - As you lift your knee, hold onto your right thigh with your hands for extra support. If you are comfortable doing so, lift your leg closer to your chest.
    - Take a pause and feel the stretch going through your thigh and hip as you breathe.
    - Slowly and gently release your right foot back to the floor and take a pause.
    - Do the same stretch on the opposite side (your left leg).

- **Breathing Technique:** Diaphragmatic Breaths

    o Put one hand on your chest and then place your other hand on your belly.

    o As you inhale slowly and deeply through your nose, feel your belly rise with your hand.

    o As you slowly exhale through your mouth, feel your belly fall with your hand as the breath leaves your body.

    o Breathe deeply into your diaphragm (the muscle below your heart and lunges). Expand your belly while inhaling and contract it as you exhale.

    o Do these diaphragmatic breaths for multiple rounds.

Phase 4: This following flow sequence allows you to begin by focusing on your upper body and then transitioning into a movement that focuses on the lower body. Earlier in the book, we mentioned props that can be used during yoga. We touched on a block, which can be helpful for the seated butterfly stretch. If you do not have one and feel comfortable with doing so, you may try it out with your feet flat on the ground. The breathing technique you will try during this phase is the lion's breath. This technique helps stimulate your throat and upper chest; it is also beneficial for relieving stress.

- **Flow Sequence:** Seated Eagle Arms to Seated Butterfly Stretch

    o Seated Eagle Arms

    - Sit in your chair with your feet flat on the ground.
    - Extend your arms directly before you, keeping them at shoulder height.
    - First, cross your right arm over your left arm, and touch your palms together if it is possible (be gentle as always).

- If you cannot touch your palms together, put the back of your right hand on top of your left palm.
- Carefully lift your elbows up; you should feel a soft stretch along your shoulders and upper back.
- Take a few deep breaths as you hold this position.
- Release the position and repeat the same stretch on the other side.

  o (2) Seated Butterfly Stretch

  - Take a seat slightly closer toward the front of your seat, keeping your feet flat on the floor.
  - Optional: if you have a yoga block, you can place this under your feet, as you can see in the image.
  - Connect the soles of your feet together and allow your knees to slowly and gently open to the sides.
  - Lightly press on your knees to deepen the stretch and sit tall.
  - If needed, hold on to your thighs for support. You can also bring your arms to a prayer position, connecting your palms together.
  - You should feel a stretch throughout your inner thighs and hips.
  - If you feel comfortable and feel like you can deepen the stretch, slightly lean forward (hinging from your hips). Ensure that your back is straight, and take it slow.
  - Remain in this position while breathing deeply and then carefully release it. Bring your feet back, remaining flat on the floor.

- **Breathing Technique**: Lion's Breath

  o Sit with good posture and put your hands on your knees.
  o Take a deep inhale through your nose.

63

o Exhale through your mouth and simultaneously stick your tongue out straight, open your eyes wide, and let out a "ha" sounds.

o Take a deep breath through your nose. As you exhale through your mouth, stick out your tongue, widen your eyes, and forcefully let out a "ha" sound.

o Repeat this breath multiple times and feel the release of tension.

Phase 5: In this final phase, we have created a more extended flow sequence. You will start with a simpler pose and slowly flow into more challenging ones. Poses from the previous chapter and this chapter have been combined. If doing a sequence of five poses seems overwhelming, feel free to start off with two and then slowly build up the flow. There is no rush when it comes to your practice. The breathing technique that you will try out in this phase, the humming bee breath, is an amazing intervention to release frustration and anger.

- **Flow Sequence:** Seated Mountain Pose to Seated Cat-Cow to Seated Warrior I to Seated Warrior II to Seated Chair Reverse Warrior

  o Seated Mountain Pose

  - Sit tall on your chair with your feet planted flat on the ground, just about hip-width apart.

  - Put your hands on your thighs with your palms facing down.

  - Lengthen your spine through good posture (sitting up straight)

  - Relax your shoulders and elongate your neck, maintaining alignment with your spine

  - Take some deep breaths (inhaling deeply from your nose and exhaling through your nose)

  - Find stability in the pose, focus on your breath, and become aware of the present moment.

- (2) Seated Cat-Cow

  - Begin by sitting tall on the chair, keeping your feet flat on the ground.
  - Put your hands on your thighs with your palms facing down.
  - Take an inhale and simultaneously arch your spine, lifting your chest forward (this is the Cow pose).
  - As you exhale, round your spine and slightly suck your stomach in, as if you are bringing your belly button inward towards your spine (this is the Cat pose).
  - Coordinate the Cow pose and Cat pose with your breath (inhaling during Cow and exhaling during Cat); smoothly slow between these two positions.
  - Feel the movement of your spin and the opening of your chest as you flow through the positions.

- (3) Seated Warrior I

  - Sit down on your chair and move closer to the front edge of your chair.
  - Slowly turn your body to the right side and move your bottom near the left edge of the chair in order to centralize yourself and create support for your right thigh (you are essentially turning sideways; you can use the back of your chair for support).
  - Keep your right hip on the chair and extend your left leg toward the floor, aligning the knee below the hip.
  - Press through the left foot, and if you'd like to deepen the pose, extend your left leg back behind you and straighten it out as much as possible (based on your own flexibility and comfort).

- Keep your arms at your hips or lengthen your body through your left arm.
- Hold this pose for several deep breaths.

- (4) Seated Warrior II

  - Sit down on your chair and move closer toward the front of your chair.
  - Put your right leg out to the right side of your chair, angling your toes straight out (your foot should be perpendicular to the chair). Bend your knee on this side.
  - Step your left foot to the left side and position your foot parallel to your chair while keeping your left leg straight.
  - You can keep your hands on your hips or reach your arms out on either side, straight out from your shoulders. They should be parallel to the floor below you.
  - Move your shoulder blades away from your ears.
  - Rotate your ribcage to the left side until your chest faces the right side, and gaze toward your right hand.

- (5) Seated Reverse Warrior

  - From the position you were in during Chair Warrior II, you can initiate this pose.
  - With your arms stretched out, inhale and slowly tilt your left arm down as your right arm goes up. You should feel a side stretch through your torso area.
  - Ensure that your neck is long and that your core muscles are engaged.

Repeat the flow on the other side, starting from the beginning

- **Breathing Technique:** Humming Bee Breath

  o Sit comfortably and close your eyes gently.

  o Put your index fingers on the cartilage of your ears and close your eyes; take a deep inhale through your nose.

  o As you exhale, make a humming sound and feel the vibration of the hum in your body.

  o Do this for a few rounds.

With poses that feel more challenging, focusing on your breath can be extra helpful. Concentrating on your breath brings you to the present moment and allows you to persevere through physical challenges. The calming effect of taking deep breaths will also help you regulate your nervous system and put you in a parasympathetic state. This state is optimal because it allows you to focus and calm down. In addition, doing exercises such as deep belly breathing leads to an increase in the flow of oxygen throughout your body and to your muscles. This allows you to endure more challenging poses for a more extended period of time. Essentially, focusing on your breath is essential with any yoga flow sequence, but it is especially important when you are trying out more challenging poses.

Furthermore, the state of meditation is simply focusing on one thing; being the observer of your thoughts and bringing yourself to the present moment. During your practice, you may find that your thoughts are all over the place. "Am I doing this right?" or "Am I doing enough?" or "What am I going to do after my practice?". Bring yourself back to this present moment and return to your breath. Observe these thoughts and let them pass, rather than attaching to them and dwelling on them. You are doing great, and this will only get easier with practice.

As you try out these more advanced poses and start to create flows, you will notice that you are becoming more aware of your mind and body. You will be more easily able to recognize tension within your body and overwhelming thoughts in your mind. When we are too distracted, it becomes hard to acknowledge the source of our mental and physical tension. Maybe sometimes you feel "off," but you are not exactly sure why. Through yoga, you have no choice but to feel present and truly reconnect with yourself. You can expand mentally and physically through this practice. When getting into more challenging poses, it is important to meet your edge, the point at which you feel challenged but can still find ease. The stretch is optimal at this point, and you are fully present. Honoring your boundaries is important; do not push yourself beyond your limits. This is a lifelong journey that will lead to self-discovery and increased awareness. The benefits of increased flexibility, mobility, independence, mental clarity, and many of the other ones that we described will come with time and consistency as you progress through your regular practice.

CHAPTER 5:

TAKE CHAIR YOGA TO THE NEXT LEVEL.

We've touched on the idea of meeting your edge during your practice. This is important because doing so will help you advance and evolve over time. What used to be a challenging pose for you will eventually be a simple pose that is a part of your daily sequence. Now, you may be wondering what kind of structure would be best for you; switching it up daily or practicing the same flow? Keeping the same sequence for a certain time period can help you master the poses within it, but you can also mix it up as well once to start to get more comfortable. In addition, you must target both your upper and lower body during your practice to prevent injuries. For this reason, it is helpful to mix up your flows so that you are strengthening a variety of muscles within your body.

In this chapter, we will give you some samples of longer flow sequences that you can incorporate into your practice. We will also talk about how you can use chair yoga to push your limits, expand your horizons, and embark on a journey of self-discovery. Your yoga practice is one that will constantly evolve with you. There is always room for expansion and innovation. We discussed various physical benefits throughout this book, but the mental benefits you will experience are just as amazing. You can experience a deeper relationship with yourself through this practice. Staying consistent with your chair yoga practice will empower you and build the trust that you have within yourself. Chair yoga is part of a new way of life, one that promotes inner peace and self-discovery. In addition, a topic that we touched on earlier in the book was chair yoga for weight loss. We will go over some chair yoga exercises that can specifically be implemented if your goal is to lose weight. We will also touch on the importance of diet in weight loss with chair yoga.

Let's get into some longer flow sequences that will encourage you to take your yoga practice to the next level. We have provided you with two different variations, containing six poses each. You may repeat your favorite sequence a few more times in order to meet the 10-minute mark. The second variation will include standing poses that were not previously mentioned, so please feel free to skip out on those if you are uncomfortable with doing them. In addition to these flow sequences, we will provide you with five new poses that are more challenging than the previous ones that we have explained. If you feel ready to take your yoga practice to the next level, these poses could be a great addition to your practice. Be gentle and slowly get into these poses; do not over-exert yourself. Safety is the number one priority when it comes to your practice, so it is important not to push beyond your limits.

- Chair Yoga Flow Sequence 1

  o Seated Mountain Pose

    - Sit tall on your chair with your feet planted flat on the ground, just about hip-width apart.
    - Put your hands on your thighs with your palms facing down.
    - Lengthen your spine through good posture (sitting up straight)

- Relax your shoulders and elongate your neck, maintaining alignment with your spine
- Take some deep breaths (inhaling deeply from your nose and exhaling through your nose)
- Find stability in the pose, focus on your breath, and become aware of the present moment.

- (2) Seated Cat-Cow Pose

  - Begin by sitting tall on the chair, keeping your feet flat on the ground.
  - Put your hands on your thighs with your palms facing down.
  - Take an inhale and simultaneously arch your spine, lifting your chest forward (this is the Cow pose).
  - As you exhale, round your spine and bring your belly button towards your spine (this is the Cat pose).
  - Coordinate the Cow pose and Cat pose with your breath (inhaling during Cow and exhaling during Cat); smoothly slow between these two positions.
  - Feel the movement of your spin and the opening of your chest as you flow through the positions.

- (3) Seated Forward Fold

  - Sit near the chair's edge while keeping your feet flat on the floor.
  - Take an inhale through your nose, lift your chest up, and lengthen your spine.
  - Exhale through your nose while hinging forward from your hips, maintaining a flat back.
  - Let your hands reach toward your thighs, shins, or feet (whatever is most comfortable for you and your level of flexibility). If possible, put

your hands on the floor (as shown in the image), but do not over-extend yourself and be very careful.

- Allow your shoulders to relax and allow your head to gently drop downward.
- Take some deep breaths and feel the stretch through the backside of your body (your legs and spine).

- (4) Chair Side Stretch

  - Sit down on the chair and keep your feet flat on the floor, maintaining good posture.
  - Interlace your fingers and bring your arms overhead (extended).
  - Take an inhale and reach upward.
  - Exhale and lean to the ride side gently; you should feel a stretch along your left waist.
  - Ensure that your shoulders are relaxed during this stretch.
  - Inhale and come back to the center.
  - Repeat this on the left side and continue to alternate sides.

- (5) Seated Eagle Arms

  - Sit in your chair with your feet flat on the ground.
  - Extend your arms directly before you, keeping them at shoulder height.
  - First, cross your right arm over your left arm, and touch your palms together if it is possible (be gentle as always).
  - If you cannot touch your palms together, put the back of your right hand on top of your left palm.

- Carefully lift your elbows up; you should feel a soft stretch along your shoulders and upper back.
- Take a few deep breaths as you hold this position.
- Release the position and repeat the same stretch on the other side.

o (6) Chair Seated Twist

- Take a seat sideways on your chair, keeping your right side closer to the backrest.
- Inhale through your nose, lengthen through your spine, and put your left hand on the outer edge of your right thigh.
- Exhale through your nose and twist your torso to the right gently. You can use your left hand to deepen the stretch as needed.
- Ensure that your head is in alignment with your spine, or slightly look over your right shoulder to deepen the stretch.
- Take deep breaths and feel the stretch; engage your core by flexing your abdominal muscles.
- Repeat this exercise on the other side by switching the positioning of your legs and arms.

- Chair Yoga Flow Sequence 2

o Seated Neck Stretch

- Begin with your feet flat on the floor, sitting tall.
- Drop your right ear onto your right shoulder while keeping your left shoulder nice and relaxed.
- If you would like to deepen the stretch, use your right to lightly press the left side of your head.

- Remain in this position for about 30 seconds to one minute while breathing deeply.
- Release the position and move your head back to the center.
- Repeat this same stretch on the opposite side.

- (2) Seated Knee Lifts

  - Sit with your feet flat on the ground, hands resting comfortably on your thighs.
  - Start by slowly lifting your right knee up towards your chest, and keep your left foot flat on the floor.
  - As you are lifting your knee, hold onto your right thigh with your hands for extra support. If you are comfortable doing so, lift your leg closer to your chest.
  - Take a pause and feel the stretch going through your thigh and hip as you breathe.
  - Slowly and gently release your right foot back to the floor and take a pause.
  - Do the same stretch on the opposite side (your left leg).

- (3) Seated Butterfly Stretch

  - Take a seat slightly closer toward the front of your seat, keeping your feet flat on the floor.
  - Optional: if you have a yoga block, you can place this under your feet, as seen in the image.
  - Connect the soles of your feet and allow your knees to slowly and gently open out to the sides.
  - Lightly press on your knees to deepen the stretch and sit tall.

- If needed, hold on to your thighs for support. You can also bring your arms to a prayer position, connecting your palms together.

- You should feel a stretch throughout your inner thighs and hips.

- If you feel comfortable and feel like you can deepen the stretch, slightly lean forward (hinging from your hips). Ensure that your back is straight, and take it slow.

- Remain in this position while breathing deeply and then carefully release it. Bring your feet back, remaining flat on the floor.

- (4) Seated Warrior II

  - Sit down on your chair and move closer toward the front of your chair.

  - Put your right leg out to the right side of your chair, angling your toes straight out (your foot should be perpendicular to the chair). Bend your knee on this side.

  - Step your left foot to the left side and position your foot parallel to your chair while keeping your left leg straight.

  - You can keep your hands on your hips or reach your arms out on either side, straight out from your shoulders. They should be parallel to the floor below you.

  - Move your shoulder blades away from your ears.

  - Rotate your ribcage to the left side until your chest faces the right side, and gaze toward your right hand.

- (5) Chair Reverse Warrior

  - From the position you were in during Chair Warrior II, you can initiate this pose.

- With your arms stretched out, inhale and slowly tilt your left arm down as your right arm goes up. You should feel a side stretch through your torso area.
- Ensure that your neck is long and that your core muscles are engaged.

- (6) Standing Chair Tree Pose (if unable to stand, do the sitting tree pose that was listed previously)

  - Stand behind your chair and place your hands on the backrest for support.
  - Keep your left foot flat on the ground as you place your right foot on your inner calf. Do not place your foot on your knee socket because this puts you at risk for dislocation.
  - Find balance within this pose and keep your posture straight.
  - If you are comfortable, place your hands at your heart center or extend them overhead, mimicking the branches of a tree.
  - Hold the pose for a few breaths before repeating it on the other side.

- Five New Challenging Poses

  - Chair Boat Pose

    - Begin by sitting on the chair.
    - Slide your bottom forward towards the front of the seat. If you can, make sure your back is not leaning on the backrest.
    - Place your hands on the seat for balance and stability.
    - Straighten your back and keep your weight on your bottom.
    - Very slightly lean back as you lift your feet off of the floor, keeping your knees bent.

- Keep your legs together as they come up. Your calves should be parallel to the floor.
- Spread your toes and press through your heels to activate your feet.
- Press your chest closer to your thighs if you feel you can do so.
- Remain in this pose for a few deep breaths.

- (2) Chair Extended Boat Pose

  - Start in the chair boat pose (as described above).
  - Slowly lean back, touching your upper back to the back of your chair.
  - Slowly extend your legs forward, squeeze your legs together, and spread your toes out.
  - Bring your belly button inwards to keep your core tight.
  - Take a few deep breaths in this pose.

- (3) Seated Figure Four

  - Begin by sitting tall in your chair, keeping your feet flat on the floor and hip distance apart.
  - Keep your left foot firmly on the ground.
  - Lift your right foot up and cross your right ankle over your right thigh. This creates a "figure four" shape.
  - Flex the right foot in order to maintain stability.
  - If you are comfortable here, gently press down on your right knee to deepen the stretch. If you feel any discomfort, do not press down.
  - Engage your core by bringing your belly button inwards and sit up tall.
  - For an even deeper stretch, hinge forward from your hips (make sure to keep your back straight and not rounded). Do not do this if it feels wrong or uncomfortable.

- Hold this pose and take a few deep breaths, feeling the stretch throughout your hip and outer thigh.
- Gently release the pose and repeat the same steps on the other side.

o (4) Box Squats

- Begin by sitting tall in your chair, keeping your feet flat on the floor and hip distance apart. Keep your chest upright.
- Inhale deeply as you engage your core muscles. Lift your arms out straight before you.
- Take an exhale as you shift your weight onto your feet and slowly stand up. As you are coming up, shift your hips forward and squeeze your glutes.
- Slowly sit back down, counting to about 3-5 seconds as you lower down.
- Once you sit down, repeat the exercise a few times.

o (5) Seated Bicycle

- Begin by sitting tall in your chair, keeping your feet flat on the floor.
- Lift your arms up and bend them towards your ears, with your fingertips essentially behind your neck.
- Keep your left leg planted on the floor and lift up your right one. At the same time, twist your upper body towards the right side. Exhale during this portion of the movement.
- Inhale as you bring your body back to the center and put your left leg down.
- Repeat this on the other side. Make sure to move in a slow and controlled manner.

- If you are up for a challenge, practice this pose while keeping both feet lifted off of the ground.
- Repeat this exercise, alternating sides, for about one minute.

These yoga flow sequences can be modified as needed. You can add or remove certain poses, or you could even combine the two flows. While it may seem challenging to remember the order of the poses, it will eventually become easier to do so. And there is no right or wrong; if you do one pose before the other, there is no harm in that. With time and as you get more comfortable with practicing, you may prefer to do flows based on what comes to mind at that moment. Speaking of advancing and evolving your practice, let's talk about using chair yoga to expand your horizons. Practicing chair yoga is an amazing opportunity to explore a non-conventional form of exercise that is gentle on your body but effective. You may have initially perceived exercise from a narrow lens, but you are now aware of a different and more accessible form of working out. The gentle stretches in chair yoga will enhance your range of motion and flexibility. You will recognize that you are breaking free from certain self-imposed limitations as you explore new poses. Maybe you never thought that you'd be able to touch the ground with your forward fold. Yet with consistent practice, you eventually do reach that point. Reaching new levels of flexibility is a rewarding part of chair yoga that you will be able to experience.

As you get comfortable with chair yoga, you may even feel more comfortable doing standing poses. This is fully up to you and should be approached slowly and gently, but maybe you'd like to try out mat yoga eventually. You may have initially started this practice in order to increase your flexibility or mobility, but as time goes on, you begin to recognize the mental benefits. The breathing exercises and mindfulness techniques that we discussed throughout this book will positively impact your mental health. Focusing on the present moment and allowing your mind to slow down will lead to discoveries within yourself. Oftentimes, we go through life thinking the same thoughts constantly. We don't always think about what we are thinking about. With these practices, you are able to take a step back and truly reflect on your mindset. This kind of introspection can lead to personal growth. With consistent practice, you may notice an increase in self-confidence within yourself and increased resilience. By overcoming the challenges of learning and practicing chair yoga, you are proving to yourself that you are strong, mentally and physically.

Another topic we mentioned in this book is using chair yoga for weight loss. This practice can benefit weight loss because it is a form of physical activity that leads you to burn calories. In addition, activating muscles through the poses can help boost your metabolism. This occurs because when you increase the amount of muscle in your body, your metabolic rate increases. Targeting various muscles through yoga also enhances the shape of your body and creates more definition.

Furthermore, yoga supports mindfulness which is beneficial for your eating habits. When you practice mindfulness during meals, you are much more aware of your hunger and fullness cues. This prevents mindless eating, an act that can easily cause you to overeat, which can eventually lead to weight gain. Along those same lines, emotional eating is a common issue that many people struggle with. During times of stress, eating food is a coping mechanism that many people lean on. By reducing stress, you will be less likely to eat emotionally or use food as a coping mechanism. Now that you know many other relaxation techniques, you have access to more tools to use during stress.

In addition to practicing chair yoga for weight loss, it is important to address nutrition. We mentioned some ways that chair yoga can help you manage your nutrition, but we will touch on some of the basics regarding weight loss. Here are three tips that you should keep in mind if you are planning on losing weight:

I. Be in a Caloric Deficit: It is important to be in a caloric deficit. This means that you are consuming fewer calories than your body burns. Controlling your portion sizes and practicing mindful eating will make it easier to be in a caloric deficit. There are certain applications where you can calculate the calories you should consume to lose weight and track your food. Still, if this is too overwhelming, there are some key things that you can focus on that will naturally put you in a caloric deficit. Increasing your intake of vegetables is a great way to stay full and not consume too many calories. In addition, make sure that you are eating protein with each meal as it keeps you full for a long time. Eating balanced meals with a source of protein, a carb, and fat will help keep you full and will help with balancing your blood sugar. Focus on eating more whole foods and less processed foods. Reducing your intake of added sugar is beneficial as well.

II. Increase Your Water Intake: Staying hydrated throughout the day is essential. Drinking water is beneficial for supporting your digestion, controlling hunger, and supporting your overall health. Oftentimes, it is easy to confuse hunger for thirst. For this reason, we must stay hydrated by regularly drinking water throughout the day. Aim to drink at least 8 cups of water per day. This can be adjusted based on your personal needs and activity levels. If you feel like drinking plain water is boring, feel free to add some lemon or fresh fruit to your water. This will add a nice flavor and possibly make you more inclined to drink water.

III. Be Consistent: Taking a long-term approach to weight loss is the best way to go about it. Weight loss is a gradual process that requires consistency and resilience. If you do not immediately see progress, do not get discouraged. It takes time to see the effects of your effort, but it will be worth it if you keep on going. It is also helpful to focus on the fact that chair yoga and a healthy diet will promote your overall well-being. Focusing on weight loss is fine, but being too attached to the potential results can make the practice unsustainable. Chair yoga is a multi-dimensional practice, and it will offer you a wide array of benefits. Being too hung up on one singular benefit can prevent you from seeing the other advantages you will experience through this practice.

In addition, here are three cardio chair yoga exercises that could help you burn some calories:

1. Seated Jumping Jacks

   a. Sit in your chair with your feet together.
   b. Move your legs out wide, extending them to the side. At the same time, raise your hands overhead.
   c. Return to the starting position quickly, lowering your arms and bringing your legs together.
   d. Repeat this jumping jack motion multiple times. Take a break and repeat. Be gentle, and do not over-exert yourself.

2. Seated High Knees

   a. Sit in your chair with your feet flat on the ground.
   b. Lift your right knee up towards your chest, and then quickly put it down as you lift your left knee up towards your chest (alternating motion).
   c. Continue to alternate between your right and left knees, as high as you comfortably can, while keeping a quick pace.
   d. Aim for 10 reps and slowly build your way up.

3. Seated Punches

a. Sit in your chair with your feet flat on the ground. Keep your hands in loose fists in front of your chest.

b. As you exhale, force your right arm forward while extending your left leg forward.

c. Take an inhale and return to your starting position.

d. As you exhale, force your left arm forward while extending your right leg forward.

e. Alternate between punches and extensions of the opposite leg, keeping a steady rhythm.

f. Repeat this for a few cycles and take a pause.

As you can see, chair yoga allows you to push your limits in many different ways. It allows you to expand your horizons and embark on a journey of self-discovery. As you continue to meet your edge during your practice, you will evolve and advance over time. Whether you choose to stick to a similar flow consistently or mix it up, you must target both the upper and lower body. This is essential in order to strengthen various muscles and prevent injuries. We've discussed how chair yoga provides an abundance of physical and mental benefits. The deeper relationship that you will create within yourself is one of the most rewarding aspects of this practice. You will build self-trust through consistent practice. Essentially, chair yoga is a new way of life in the most beautiful and expansive way possible. We provided you with poses and sequences that will allow you to take your practice to the next level. Finally, we covered chair yoga for weight loss and other factors that should be considered if this is your main goal. Remember that it is essential to approach your practice from a place of gentleness. Be bold, but always put your safety first, and do not push beyond your limits.

CONCLUSION:
CHAIR YOGA FAQ

1) Question: Is chair yoga really suitable for everyone?

Answer: Yes, chair yoga can be done by nearly anyone. This form of exercise is designed to be accessible to people of all fitness levels. It is especially beneficial for seniors over 60 and people with physical limitations who are looking for a gentle form of exercise. It can be modified as needed to meet the needs of the practitioner. It is safe for seniors above 60, but it is essential to talk to your doctor or primary healthcare provider before starting any new exercise programs.

2) Question: How often should I practice chair yoga, and for how long?

Answer: Consistency is the most important aspect when it comes to chair yoga. So if you only have 5 minutes to practice one day, that is still better than doing nothing. Ideally, starting with 5-10 minute sessions a few times a week and then gradually increasing the duration is the best way to go about it. As you get more comfortable with the practice, you can exercise for longer. Listen to your body and create a routine that works for you and allows you to be consistent.

3) Question: How can I stay consistent with my chair yoga practice?

Answer: As we previously mentioned, start with shorter sessions and then gradually work your way up. Even just a few minutes will be beneficial for your mind and body. Another helpful thing is to make your practice a part of your morning or nightly routine. For instance, maybe after breakfast, you decide that this is the time that you do your practice. You could also set reminders on your phone or place sticky notes to remind you to practice. Make sure to be flexible with yourself and mix up your flows so you do not get bored. Celebrate your achievements along the way because this will help motivate you to continue practicing.

4) Question: Can chair yoga help with pain management?

Answer: Yes, chair yoga can be a helpful tool for pain management. The gentle stretches promote flexibility and relaxation, which can lead to a decrease in tension within the body. Breathing and relaxation techniques can also help decrease pain. As always, it is important to consult with your provider before using a new form of exercise to manage pain.

5) Question: Can chair yoga help improve balance and prevent falls in seniors?

Answer: Yes, chair yoga is a great way to improve stability and balance in seniors. The movements help strengthen the core, which is essential for maintaining balance. As we mentioned earlier in the book, chair yoga helps improve proprioception which can reduce the risk of falls. In addition, yoga exercises that involve shifting weight in the body help improve balance.

6) Question: Is it necessary to warm up before starting your chair yoga practice?

Answer: Chair yoga is a gentle practice, but warming up before starting can be helpful. Starting off with simple movements such as neck stretches, shoulder rolls, and wrist circles can be beneficial to help warm up your body. Warming up supports flexibility and circulation, reducing the risk of injury.

7) Question: Can chair yoga help improve sleep quality in seniors?

Answer: Yes, chair yoga can help improve sleep quality in seniors. With breathing exercises, relaxation techniques, and gentle movements, you experience calming effects on your mind and body. It can be beneficial to practice yoga before bedtime to relax and prepare for a peaceful night of sleep.

8) Question: Are there chair yoga poses that can help relieve back pain?

Answer: Yes, there are many different chair yoga poses that can be helpful in relieving back pain. For instance, seated spinal twists and seated cat-cow stretches can improve spine flexibility and potentially relieve pain. As always, it is important to consult with a healthcare provider if you'd like to implement these techniques in order to manage your back pain.

9) Question: Can chair yoga be helpful for seniors with arthritis?

Answer: Yes, chair yoga can benefit individuals struggling with arthritis or joint stiffness. These gentle movements can assist with increasing your joint mobility and reduce stiffness. If your arthritis makes certain poses challenging, you can modify them to accommodate your needs.

10) Can chair yoga be done at home if seniors cannot attend classes?

Of course! All exercises discussed in this book can be practiced from the comfort of your home. We have given you an abundance of poses that you can incorporate into your at-home yoga practice. In addition, there are many videos online that directly guide you through yoga flow sequences. As we have mentioned, ensuring safety is your top priority when practicing chair yoga at home or in a studio.

ABOUT THE AUTHOR

Arnold Barber is the author of Chair Yoga for Seniors Over 60: 10 Minutes a Day to Enhance Flexibility, Balance, and Mobility - A Quick and Simple Step-by-Step Guide for Weight Loss and Improved Independence.

Arnold Barber is a reputable author as he is deeply passionate about the subject of chair yoga for the elderly. His enthusiasm for this topic is evident in the comprehensive and practical approach he takes in the book.

Arnold Barber is an experienced chair yoga practitioner who has dedicated several years to the study and practice of this form of yoga specifically designed for the elderly. His experience and knowledge shines through in the book, providing readers with valuable insights and guidance.

Arnold Barber personally understands the challenges and obstacles seniors can face when it comes to flexibility, balance and mobility. He successfully dealt with these issues using chair yoga and changed his life. In his book, he aims to set readers on the same path to improved physical well-being and independence.

Arnold Barber's motivation for writing this book stems from his desire to share his experience and knowledge with others. He recognizes the transformative potential of chair yoga for seniors and wants to empower people to improve their overall quality of life through practice.

Made in United States
Troutdale, OR
09/20/2023

13056433R00053